Paleo Diet

A quick beginner guide

By Rick Paul

Table of Contents

Introduction

I want to thank you and congratulate you for downloading the book, Paleo Diet.

This book contains proven steps and strategies about Paleo diet. This book is an excellent guide for people who want to know everything there is to know about the Paleo Diet. This Book is the Ultimate Guidelines for a beginner.

The Paleo diet is a low carb diet, with a high amount of protein and a lot of vegetables. This diet is sometimes referred to as the "Caveman Diet" because it is basically anything that was eaten by a caveman. This diet is so effective because it forces your body to burn fats for energy, instead of glucose from carbs.

If your goal is to lose weight, keep it off, and increase energy levels, you need to eat all natural, non processed foods like the caveman did. The caveman didn't have the technology to grow grains or make dairy products, so why would we eat them?.Adapting the caveman diet will not only help you live a healthy and fulfilling life but you will also be able to cut fat and look the way you've always wanted.

This book will provide all information needed to implement the Paleo Diet in your life.I will discuss about the Paleo,the benefits of Paleo,What you can eat when on a Paleo diet, **What Food Should You Avoid**.I will help you implement the Paleo Diet.

You will get exact and reliable information in regards to the topic and issue covered. The book is sold with the information that the publisher is not necessary to render accounting, officially acceptable, or otherwise, professional services. If information is necessary, legal or acceptable, an experienced individual in the profession should be ordered.

Thanks again for downloading this book, I hope you enjoy it!

Chapter 1 What is paleo ?

The Paleo diet is a very healthy way that you can eat because it is the one kind of food approach that works with your genetics to help you to stay slim, strong and active. Studies in biology, biochemistry, Ophthalmology, Dermatology, and many other specialties have determined that it is our new nutrition, which is full of refined food, unhealthy fats and sugar, that is at the source of progressive diseases, such as obesity, malignancy, diabetes, heart disease, and many others.

The Paleolithic food plan is a new, healthy plan that is based on the food consumed in Paleolithic times. It is based on several key ideas, including: 1. Social heredities have barely improved since the beginning of agriculture, which was about fifty thousand years back at the end of the Paleolithic age; 2. The new persons adjust to the food or diets of the Paleolithic time and; 3. It is probable for new science to determine what such a food plan consisted of.

The people who are familiar with the Paleo diet say that the modern people who exist on ordinary food, the same types believed to be consumed by Paleolithic hunter-gatherers, are mainly free from disease and have found that eating Paleolithic food has shown better health results when compared to other largely-recommended food plans.

The Paleo Diet Method

The Paleo food, which is the genuine term for food in the Paleolithic Diet method, consists of the types of food contained in the diet that the Paleolithic man would have had in prehistoric years.

There's no question that, as time has progressed onwards, knowledge and cooking procedures have significantly improved since the age of our forefathers. They would have to actually go out and search in the world for the foods for their diets. Today, we simply take a quick trip to the grocery store, where we're met with a large selection of a variety of foods that have been properly treated and prepared to eat.

The problem with this is that, while these changes have happened, we've polluted the nutrition of our regular food and are missing out on the essential elements in our food that nature intended for us to have. We've added to the convenience of food, but this has happened at the cost of nutrition.

The idea of the Paleolithic food is to go back to the natural food of prehistoric times. When accepting this dieting method, you choose to forgo all of the new types of foods that you find at the supermarket and instead focus on a diet that is natural and balanced. Basically, if it was accessible thousands of years ago, it's beneficial to have in a meal that you are planning.

Purpose of the Paleo Diet

The Paleo diet is created with the knowledge that people's figures used to be developed through the largely dependable food bases that were accessible to prehistoric collectors. Over time, the body adjusted to this diet and responded to it optimally. Preservatives and other cultivated products were presented comparatively recently in man's history, and are detrimental to the body because they are not as nutritionally valuable as the traditional foods of the Paleolithic age.

Chapter 2   The benefits of a Paleo diet

One of the mistaken beliefs about the Paleo diet is that it's focused on proteins with fat. Combine that with the improved health and increased nutrient absorption that happens through the avoidance of irritating grains and legumes, and you get a very balanced diet. You will be astonished that anyone can have all of the compulsory nutrients that are found in animal, seafood and plant created diets. Here you can see 10 Paleo diet benefits.

10 Paleo diet benefits

1. Well-developed Brain

One of the best bases of protein and fat recommended by the Paleo diet originates from icy water fish; preferably wild-caught salmon. Other bases of omega 3 fatty acids are found in pasture-raised herbs and seed.

2. Develop all Essential Vitamins & Minerals

The Paleo nutrition recommends consumption of multicolored food. Root vegetables are a great part of the diet and it's able to offer a variability of vegetables, contingent on the seasons.

The different types of vegetarians are in need of the nutrients they include! By eating the colorful foods, you confirm that you are getting all of your vitamins.

3. Good Digestion and Absorption

The Paleo Diet proposes the consumption of foods that you've acquired the skill to digest rapidly over thousands of ages. There are no questions whether or not you might bear starch or grass-fed complaints. Your ancestors lived and prospered off these diets.

4. A Smaller amount Allergies

The Paleo Diet suggests that you avoid foods that are well-known to be allergy-inducing in some societies. Some persons are incapable of processing seeds and dairy, which is why the Paleo Diet strongly suggests you limit these diets to a minimum every month.

Persons often gather that the Paleo Diet doesn't have whole grains. The reality is just that grains are not the greatest foods for energy, so we avoid them most of the time, but not continuously. If you are an athlete, you may need to consume a single cup of oats before you compete.

5. Decrease Infection

Studies propose that inflammation may be an important factor for heart disease. What you should know about the Paleo Diet is that a lot of the foods have anti-inflammatory agents so you will be reducing your danger.

The greater focus on omega 3 fatty acids is one of the benefits of those foods is that they are anti-inflammatory.

6. Extra Energy

Ever wonder why energy juices have become so standard in the last decade? It's because everybody's food sucks!

A classic American mealtime consists of a honey, coffee coupled with a muffin or bagel with cream cheese. Not only does this eventually lead to two kinds of diabetes and insulin opposition, but also it won't even keep you satiated. With the Paleo Diet, you intentionally select the correct foods all the time.

7. Weight Loss

The Paleo Diet is a low-carb diet by design. Just removing preserved nutrients radically decreases your carb consumption and results in weight loss.By avoiding carbs, you will evade an unwelcome fat increase, which is often produced by these extra carbs.

8. Decrease Danger of Disease

The Paleo Diet's main focus is to escape diets that can potentially harm your health. The Paleo diet makes it easy to avoid bad foods by giving you a simple blueprint; only eat what a caveman would be able to eat.

When this is followed, it will ensure that you eat whole foods, and limit your danger for infection by escaping the foods recognized to originate them.

9. Shrink Person's Fat Cells

Most people don't fully realize that fat cells shrink and increase based on your food. A slim person does not have less fat cell, they just have smaller cells. A way to make your fat cells smaller is to select good fats and limit your carb eating. All elements the Paleo Diet proposes. Good fats are collected within your chambers and are readily accessible for energy when someone is insulin deficient.

10. Detox Effects

When you stop consuming things that sabotage your health, such as caffeine, refined sugar, trans fats, gluten, and more, you are giving your body a break. You'll be purging your body of all the built-up toxic foods. We call this a detox. Many Paleo Dieters report that they feel lighter and more focused after just a couple of weeks. After you've had your detox, your cheat meal won't have the same satisfying effect as when you were addicted. In fact, you'll experience negative side effects immediately when you have your cheat meal. You'll suffer from diarrhea, headaches and instant bloating. This will help you to be less likely to implement cheat meals and allow you to cut out processed foods for good.

Chapter 3   What you can eat when on a Paleo diet

Many people get confused when I say that eating fat is very healthy for you. Some cannot even accept the fact that this is true. But the truth is, eating fats is very healthy for you. It has several benefits like improving bones, liver health, healthy lungs, immune system, and promoting a healthy brain. Here you can see some Paleo diet food list.

Paleo Diet Food List

Meat

Goat, sheep, horse, wild boar, pork, rabbit, lamb, beef, bison.

Game meat

Bear, moose, woodcock, elk, duck, rabbit, reindeer, wild turkey, deer, pheasant.

Fish

Salmon, trout, bass, sole, haddock, turbot, tilapia, cod, flatfish, grouper, mackerel, anchovy, tuna, walleye, halibut.

Fats

avocado oil, olive oil, avocados, coconut oil, clarified butter (ghee), lard, tallow, butter, duck fat, veal fat, lamb fat, fatty fishes, nut butters, nut oils (walnut, macadamia), milk coconut.

Paleo Diet Seafood

Down in New Orleans and want to have a gumbo? With the Paleo diet, change it out for shrimp. Want to enjoy a meal at the Red Lobster? Check out the loads of alternative seafood you can enjoy on the paleo diet.

Crab, Crawfish, Crayfish, Clams, Shrimp, lobster, Scallops, Oysters, Mushrooms, Button mushroom, Portobello, Oyster Mushroom, Chanterelle, Crimini, Porcini

Paleo Diet Root vegetable

The Paleo Diet is comprised of many root vegetables. Almost all vegetables are considered in the Paleo diet as being healthy, but you still need to be aware of the starch content. Root vegetables with the maximum starch content – such as potatoes and jams - are likely to have a lower nutritional value, depending on the quantity of starches and sugars they have. Although they are not good for you, they're not completely off-limits. The following chart shows some of the accepted Paleo Diet Root vegetables:

Asparagus	Avocado
Artichoke hearts	Carrots
Brussels sprouts	Spinach
Broccoli	Zucchini
Celery	Cabbage

Cauliflower	Eggplant
Green Onions	Peppers (All Kinds)
Parsley	Coconut oil

Contrary to popular belief, fats in food don't make you overweight – carbohydrates do and the typical American food has a lot of them. Natural oils and body fats are your body's desired method of producing energy so it's important to provide your body with what it's requesting! Below are some of the greatest kinds of foods that contain paleo oils and fats that you can provide your body with needed sustained energy.

Paleo Diet Nuts

Our favorite nuts! (Does that sound bad?) Nuts are definitely Paleo. Be wary though as cashews are full of fat and so delicious that it can be easy to eat a whole jar in one meeting. If you're trying to lose weight, limit the serving of nuts you are allowed and stick to it!

You can also try a decent pecan/walnut/almond nut mix as well. The following chart shows some of the good Paleo Diet nuts:

Almonds	Cashews
Hazelnuts	Pecans
Pine Nuts	Paleo Diet Fruits
Pumpkin Seeds	Sunflower Seeds
Macadamia Nut	Walnuts

Paleo Diet fruits

Paleo Diet fruits are not only attractive but also they are very good for you. Paleo accepted fruits are those that contain great quantities of fructose that is much more preferred over HFCS (high-fructose corn syrup) – but it is still sugar. If you're looking to lose extra weight on the Paleo Diet, you'll need to limit the fruits and focus more on the root vegetables allowed on the Paleo diet. However, feel free to enjoy 1-3 portions of fruit a day. Check out this list of Paleo Diet fruits and see if you're not starving by the time you get to the bottom! (We'll admit, we're partial to the blackberries).

Apple	Avocado
Blackberries	Papaya
Peaches	Plums
Mango	Blueberries
Lychee	Figs
Grapes	Lemon
Strawberries	Watermelon

Oranges	Bananas
Raspberries	Cantaloupe
Tangerine	Pineapple

List of Foods Not Acceptable on the Paleo Diet

This is an essential list of food that is not acceptable on the Paleo Diet. It's very difficult to let these types of foods go once you start out on your Paleo food journey, but as you continue you will find that it gets easier and you will discover many Paleo food alternatives to replace your old favorites. The first few weeks will be hard, but if you make the switch, it'll be very beneficial to you. We have the ability. Here's the final list of foods that are not acceptable on the Paleo Diet.

- No fast food
  (candy, , ice cream ,crackers, snack foods)

- No Beans
  (lima beans, dark beans, peanuts, baked beans)

- No Sugar or Synthetic Sugar
  (Splenda, pure cane, corn syrup, honey, maltodextrin, Equal, Stevia, agave nectar, syrup, etc.)

- No Starches
  (wheat goods, corn goods, pasta, cereals, rice, oatmeal, bread)

- No Dairy

- No Alcohol

Chapter 4   Paleo exercise

In modern life, we use lots of instruments and machines for exercise to keep our body fit and to make body muscles. But it is possible to make a fit body and impressive muscles just with some movements called paleo exercise. This is the type of movements that the ancient cavemen did perform to survive against adverse and unpredictable environment and to protect themselves from wild animals. There are several steps of paleo exercise. They are discussed below:

1. Warm-up: Before starting any exercise, you need to warm up your body muscles. Otherwise, muscles can be injured during exercise. For this, you can use a treadmill or simply can walk or run for several minutes, can jump, and do some movements of every part of the body.

2. Squatting: Squatting is the bending of the knee and hips keeping the back straight. You can take some weight on your shoulder and hold the weight when squatting but it is not very much necessary. You can also perform simple squatting without any weight.

3. Bending: You'll have to hold tow, simple weights in your two hands and bend side to side. At least 10 times bending is needed in each side.

4. Lunging: Take a barbell on your shoulder, then step up on a chair or bench alternating the legs in every step. Do at least 20 times.

5. Pushing: Stand up and hold a cable or elastic band. Then push forward like punching. Do it 20 times with each arm. Switch the arm and repeat it.

6. Pulling: Just do the reverse movement of pushing. Hold the cable or elastic band and pull it down instead of pushing.

7. Twisting: Now hold the cable with both arms, keep the arms straight and twist in both sides. Do it 10 times in each side.

8. Lifting weight: Lift any heavy things. It can be anything like rock, tree, tires or can use dumbbell and barbell. When you lift any weight from the ground, there is a possibility to injure the veins of waist. So, be careful about this or use waistband when lifting any heavy weight.

9. Dips or pushup: Dips is a very useful Paleo exercise which affects on chest, shoulder, back and arms. No additional weight is required for dips. Just use the body weight. Pushup or dips is raising lowering the body, placing two hands on the ground.

10. Resting: In all exercise programs, resting is a most necessary thing. Our body muscles need rest to make the proper development and to maintain fitness. So, it is generally advised to do exercise in every alternative day.

Also, it is to mention that during exercise, it is needed to drink a lot of water because during exercise, our body temperature becomes high and water controls the temperature inside. So, after completing each set of exercise, drinking water is must.

The basic goal of paleo exercise is to improve body strength and fitness. Paleo diet is also helpful to keep the fitness during paleo workout.

Chapter 5   Top Paleo habits

Human beings are creatures of habit. Most things you do on a daily basis, you do automatically. Our brain tends to create habits so we can focus on the things in our life that really matter. For example, when you are driving a car you are doing this effortlessly (most of the time). You are not thinking about all the little steps you are taking. You just step into your car, turn on the engine, and go. And all this while talking with the person next to you. Why is that? This is because we created this habit by repeating it often. If you had to think consciously about every little step you needed to take, you wouldn't be able to focus on other things.

The same thing goes with your diet. Most of the time, we eat the same thing, the same amount, and at the same time every day. This helps us to focus on the important tasks in our life and not on our food.

Replace Your Food One Step at a Time

When you want to implement the Paleo Diet, it is very important to do this one step at a time. It is too difficult to change your whole diet overnight. You can try it, but most of the time, you will fall back because it's too much to digest at once. It's like the saying eat the elephant piece by piece'. It is important to replace your bad foods with good foods. Here is a 5-step action plan for how to implement the Paleo Diet immediately.

1.Start with the beverages

The easiest and most important thing you can change overnight is replacing all your beverages with water and green tea. A lot of the daily sodas and juices we consume contain a lot of added sugars, toxins, and empty calories. The best thing you can do is to avoid these beverages and consume water or green tea instead.You will notice that you are going to feel much better because you are getting rid of all of those artificial drinks. If you really don't like the taste of plain water or green tea, you can be creative with it. Start mixing water with fresh fruit. This will give you the sweet taste while drinking a lot of water.

2.Replace Sugar with Honey

Honey is Paleo, sweet and a lot healthier than sugar. So, if you really have a sweet tooth and can't possibly find a way to get rid of sweets, I highly recommend that you replace your sugar with honey.

3.Replace the Bad Carbohydrates with Paleo Substitutes

Some of the toughest things to remove from our diet are processed carbs. I always loved potatoes, pastas, and bread. We ate these things a lot at home and when I started to change my diet, I couldn't find a way to get rid of these carbs. I tried to eat more vegetables, but it did not do the trick for me. The one thing that helped me to control my carb cravings were Paleo substitutes. Paleo substitutes taste just like your favorite carbs, but are healthy and Paleo.

4.Start Eating Grass-Fed Meat, Fish, and Eggs

If you didn't already, start eating grass fed meat, fish, and eggs. You can choose which meats, fish, or eggs you'll eat, but it is important to eat them all in a good balance. The best way to implement this is by trying a new meat, fish, and egg every day and writing down which ones you really like. Fine-tune this until you have a perfect mix you like

5. Only Keep Paleo Foods at Home

Start throwing away (or giving away if you think throwing away food is a waste) all the non-Paleo foods. Also, start buying Paleo foods only. This will help you stick with the diet when you are having a hard time. When you start to implement the Paleo Diet, it will come as a willpower challenge to stay away from pastas, bread, or other things you really love. If you keep them at home, you will most likely eat them, even if you weren't intending to eat them at first. So get rid of these foods.

Chapter 6   Paleo and Weight Loss

Here are a number of great tips of how to lose weight on the Paleo diet:

1. Keep your diet simple.

One of the reasons the Paleo diet is so helpful with weight loss is due to its ability to help you decrease the number of calories that you consume unknowingly. Studies have demonstrated that eating smaller portions leads to consuming less food, which in turn helps you to avoid having an excess of calories.

2. Be sure to eat enough.

Numerous Paleo newbies think that less food is always better when it comes to losing weight. This belief causes you to deprive your body of the calories and nutrients needed to be at your best and reasons further pressure. Lessening your caloric intake lowers your latent metabolic rate, which can cause you to actually gain weight. No matter what diet you choose, starving yourself should never be an option. Calories are a vital part of our existence.

3. Eat enough carbs to provide for your activity level.

Carbohydrate intake is completely different, and I've seen people who do fairly well on a low carb diet, while others crash and burn. Typically, the main issue is the quantity and level of activity the person is involved in, as many of my patients trying to lose weight are taking part in challenging strength exercise machines, such as Crossfit, or spend many hours at the local fitness center.

4. Change throughout the day.

Being too inactive can decrease the benefits of your exercise program and prevent weight loss. If you work in an office, travel by car and watch too many hours of television at night, it's not hard to understand how you could spend a large portion of your waking hours sitting on your bottom. Also, a workout alone isn't enough to counteract the damaging effects of a sedentary lifestyle. When it comes to weight loss, having energy throughout the whole day, and not just during the 60 minutes you work at the gymnasium, is a vital part of a healthy routine.

5. Never do it by yourself.

One of the toughest parts of losing weight is trying to do it all by yourself. Creating major life changes without any help from friends is not only difficult, but often unmanageable. Asking friends or family to inspire you, or even make changes along with you, can significantly increase your achievement in any major life change, specifically the change to a Paleo diet. You can share plans, arrange partner challenges, and inspire each other on your trip to good health.

6. Discourse your entire life, not just food and application.

Focus on managing stress using mind-body methods, like meditation or yoga. Think about using shopping and meal plans to help you decrease the stress that comes along with starting a big life change. Spend time with friends and family, and gather support in your weight loss efforts. You'll be more likely to lose weight and keep it off for the long haul. And you'll really be able to enjoy living your life.

The Positive weight loss isn't about the number of calories in your low-carb tortillas, or "counteracting" each treat with an hour of sweating it out at the gym. Striving to starve your body into shape without considering your natural metabolic challenges and food desires will be unsuccessful and will not bring the desired results. The way to permanent weight loss is mending the harm brought to your metabolism and hormonal systems from the toxic modern food environment; a ketogenic Paleo diet gives your body the opportunity to heal itself, making a solid foundation for your lasting fitness, not a temporary change to your tie size.

Conclusion

Thank you again for buying this book!

I hope this book was able to help you to know about Paleo Diet.

Finally, if you enjoyed this book, then I'd like to ask you for a favor, would you be kind enough to leave a review for this book on Amazon? It'd be greatly appreciated!

Thank you and good luck